ULRIKE NARINS

Folk Dance Musings

How folk dancing can enrich all aspects of your life

This book was professionally typeset on Reedsy.
Find out more at reedsy.com

"So many dances, so little time"

- unknown

Contents

1

Introduction

W elcome to *Folk Dance Musings*! I'm Ulrike Narins, and I am so excited to share my passion for folk dancing with you.

In this book, you'll discover my journey into the world of folk dancing and the many adventures I've had along the way. Over the years, I've been continually amazed by the countless benefits of folk dancing, and I'm writing this book so that you don't have to wait years to uncover these wonderful aspects for yourself.

But before we dive in, let me explain what international folk dancing is, in case you're unfamiliar. It encompasses dances from around the world, representing various countries and cultures. The dances themselves take many forms—circle dances, line dances, set dances, couple dances, mixers, progressive couple dances, and circle dances without hand-holding.

There are just three simple rules for folk dancing:

1. Don't harm yourself.

2. Don't harm others.
3. Have fun!

One of my favorite sayings in folk dancing is, "There are no mistakes, only solos!"

You'll also notice that I mention my son Lothar quite often. His name is pronounced with a silent "h." And when I talk about "Changs," I'm referring to "Changs International Folk Dancers", the longest continuously active folk dance group in the United States, based in San Francisco, California. If you're curious about a dance I mention, you can easily look it up on YouTube by typing in the dance name followed by the word "dance" to see it in action.

Lastly, I want to share that I am currently finishing my term as President of the Folk Dance Federation of Northern California.

2

My First Steps

I'd like to share a bit about my journey as a folk dancer and how my experiences and outlook have transformed over time. I came to international folk dancing somewhat late, as I wasn't even aware of its existence before 2008. Growing up in Austria, I was only familiar with "Volkstanz," which to me meant "Laendler," women in Dirndls, men in Lederhosen, and music played on zithers and accordions—a tradition I never found particularly appealing.

It wasn't until I moved to San Francisco in my thirties that things began to shift. When my son went to college, he spent his junior year in Germany, where he developed an interest in folk dancing. Upon his return, he introduced me to it and took me to the folk dance group near our home, Changs International Folk Dancers, that had warmly welcomed him. I was immediately captivated by the music, representing so many different countries, and the dances with their unfamiliar names. The group embraced me with open arms as well. At first, I danced mostly behind the line, carefully learning the steps. It wasn't as easy as it might have been when I was younger, and I often thought that more emphasis should be placed on getting the steps exactly right.

However, as the dances became more instinctive, I found myself fully immersed in the joy of moving with the music. My focus began to expand beyond the steps, and I grew more aware of the warmth, tolerance, and inclusivity that defined this community. It touched my heart. I also began to appreciate how mistakes were treated—not as something to be criticized, but as part of the learning process, with everyone included regardless. It was then that I realized I had found my village, my tribe, a place where I truly belonged.

There is one person I must mention: Laila Messer. Without her, I wouldn't be dancing today. She welcomed my son, Lothar, to Changs with such kindness that he returned and encouraged me to give it a try.

Reflecting on my journey, two important things stand out. First, my own shift in perspective has made me more tolerant of those with less inclusive views, knowing they too might change. And second, a warm and welcoming atmosphere is key to encouraging new dancers to return and become part of the community.

3

Including Folk Dancing when Traveling

I 've had the pleasure of dancing in many different places. In South Bend, Indiana, I enjoyed easy dances with a welcoming group, and in New York City's Central Park, I had the chance to meet Moshe Eskayo, a renowned choreographer of Israeli dances. While dancing in Canada, I discovered that some groups take breaks during the summer or winter months, and I couldn't help but wonder how folk dancers manage to go so long without dancing! Every now and then, however, a truly remarkable experience comes along, like the one I had in Vienna, Austria.

In Vienna, I stumbled upon a Bulgarian group that had combined their intermediate and performance-level dancers for their final evening before the summer break. Despite the language barrier—they welcomed me in a mix of broken German and English—once the dancing started, everything was in Bulgarian. I didn't understand a word, but it was thrilling to simply follow along by watching, instead of listening for instructions. We began with a brief warm-up using ballet movements, which was relatively easy to follow, but things quickly became much more challenging. We danced continuously for 45 minutes—all fast-paced dances! Imagine dancing "Eleno Mome" or "Oj Dimitro Le" for that long without a break! Most of the dances were unfamiliar to me, so I had to stay completely focused. Even the dances I thought I knew were performed differently than what I was used to at Changs, so I never had a chance to relax. Twice I tried to sit and rest, but each time someone pulled me back into the line. To my surprise, I made it through the 45 minutes without collapsing, and the experience was exhilarating! In the break the group sang a beautiful Bulgarian birthday song for one of the dancers. After the break, the pace slowed down a bit. At one point, we danced "T' Smidje," a couple mixer to the tune of "Drunken Sailor," which allowed us to skip the long introduction of the original piece and start dancing sooner.

During a visit to my son in Berlin, we attended a folk dance group that was quite different from the ones I had danced with in the U.S. The group was younger, with more men than women. Although they more or less ignored Lothar and me, we still enjoyed the dancing. At one point, they announced "Mori Shej," and I was excited to finally recognize a dance. But no, it wasn't the same at all—the music and the steps were entirely different! This reminded me of the advice our teacher at Changs, Craig Blackstone, always gives: when dancing with groups outside your home group, never try to lead—just follow along with how the dances are done there. When in Rome, do as the Romans do!

Dancing with different groups around the world allows you to connect with locals in a way that goes beyond the typical tourist experience, and it broadens your folk dance horizons. Another joy of dancing while traveling is bringing a new dance back home to share with your own group. Whenever I've done that, I've developed a special connection to the dance, making it all the more meaningful.

4

Finding Folk Dance Venues in Rural Japan

I'd like to continue the theme of dancing away from home. Whenever I've looked for a place to dance, whether in the U.S. or Europe, my first step has always been an online search. Usually, I'd find listings with details about the types of dances, schedules, and contact information. From there, I'd simply show up at the address on the designated day, ready to dance.

However, my experience in Japan in 2016 was quite different. My son, Lothar, and I had the unique opportunity to live for six months at a Buddhist temple in a remote part of Yamaguchi Prefecture. Naturally, I couldn't imagine going that long without dancing, so I asked around for advice. I was told to contact a Japanese folk dancer, who often brings foreign dance instructors on tours through Japan. I assumed she would direct me to a website where I could find all the information I needed. But that wasn't the case. Instead, she reached out to her network and eventually connected me with someone in Himeji, who then introduced me to Mr. Hagi in Yamaguchi Prefecture. He was involved with several local dance circles near the temple.

Mr. Hagi expressed some concerns, both his own and those of the local dancers, about the potential awkwardness of including a foreigner in their dance circles. He asked several questions:

- Was the American á man or a woman?
- Did this person want to join regular dance groups, practice sessions, or participate in parties and workshops?
- What days and times would work best—mornings, afternoons, or evenings? And what about weekends or public holidays?
- (And most importantly) How well does the person speak Japanese, since no one there speaks English?
- Would transportation be an issue? (He offered to assist with that.)

After a good deal of indirect communication, I eventually began corresponding with Mr. Hagi directly, working with my Japanese tutor to ensure my responses were respectful and clear. My only goal was to dance with other folk dancers, despite the logistical challenges.

A few days after we arrived at the temple, Mr. Hagi came for an introductory meeting. The head monk announced that the folk dance group had arrived, and Lothar and I were invited to join them. It turned out that several people had come, and they brought us gifts. I later learned that they were board members of the Yamaguchi Folk Dance Federation, including the president, and some had traveled quite a distance for this meeting. Though I couldn't understand everything that was said, I gathered that there was some discussion about whether we were skilled enough dancers to fit in and how they should assess this. But whenever we mentioned the name of a folk dance, the person we were speaking with would light up, and we knew we shared a common passion.

In the end, it was decided that Mr. Hagi would pick us up a few days later for our first dance evening with one of the local dance circles. Persistence certainly pays off!

More to come in the next chapter about my folk dance adventures in Japan.

<h1 style="text-align:center">5</h1>

Folk Dancing in Rural Japan: The Beginnings

I'd like to share some of the experiences my son Lothar and I had with the weekly dance circles we attended during our six-month stay at a Buddhist temple in Japan. Initially, Mr. Hagi drove us to the dances twice a week, but over time, he taught us the way, and we began driving ourselves using one of the temple's cars. Navigating to locations in Japan proved more challenging than in Europe or the U.S.

To prepare, I studied dance-related vocabulary so I could understand the instructions during lessons. But when I heard Mr. Hagi teaching, I realized that all the Japanese terms I had carefully memorized weren't as useful as I had hoped. Many of the dance terms were English expressions pronounced with a Japanese accent. For example, "hop step" became "hoppu steppu," "quick quick slow" was "kuiku kuiku suroh," and "two step" was "tsuh steppu," meaning step-together-step.

We did our best to be respectful and integrate into the group. We bowed often and deeply. Most of the dancers were older women, with only a few men, and nearly all of them were skilled dancers who picked up complex steps and sequences quickly. At first, the dancers were shy around us.

During progressive couple dances, some women would wave us on to the next partner rather than dancing with us. But as time passed, we were increasingly accepted. They started bringing us small gifts, and we reciprocated by offering chocolates. By the time we left Japan, we had grown quite fond of each other, and our farewell was deeply emotional.

Every month, the temple hosted an "open house" where neighbors and friends would gather for lunch and special events, and local farmers and merchants would offer goods and services. During our stay, the folk dancers were invited to perform at these gatherings in front of the Buddha. Dancing together on the tatami mats in our stockings or socks felt like a special experience for everyone involved.

As people grew more comfortable around us, we began asking them to teach us some Japanese dances to bring back to our group in San Francisco. Although they didn't typically dance many Japanese dances, they were eager to share a few with us. In turn, they asked us to teach them some of the dances from our repertoire. As a result, the Blackstone Jig, choreographed by our teacher at Changs, Craig Blackstone, has now spread to three continents: North America, Europe, and Asia.

One memorable moment occurred when Mr. Hagi announced that we would be dancing the "keosu mikusa," which we recognized as the Chaos Mixer. However, instead of embracing the usual unpredictability of the dance, he meticulously explained how the couples should position themselves and move to the next partner. Lothar and I were taken by surprise and struggled not to laugh. It was clear that, for them, the name of the dance was just a series of sounds. Afterward, I explained the meaning of the name and how we dance it in the U.S.

The dancers had been quite serious during our sessions, but as we all became more relaxed, Lothar and I started dancing more expressively. To our delight, we noticed that the Japanese dancers began to have more fun, too. After we returned to the U.S., I received a heartfelt email from Mr. Hagi, expressing how much our presence had inspired his dancers to embrace a more joyful, youthful style of dancing.

6

Folk Dancing in Rural Japan: Surprises

In addition to the weekly dance circles, we were invited to participate in a monthly workshop held in the town of Ube, where a dedicated group of dancers gathered for a full day of dancing. Typically, Mr. Hagi or another member of the group would teach a new dance. Once everyone was ready, Mr. Hagi would record the teacher explaining the dance steps, followed by a recording of the group performing the dance. Over the course of the day, about eight dances were taught in this way. Mr. Hagi generously shared many of these videos with me, which have become cherished memories as well as valuable references for reviewing the dance steps.

During one of the workshops, we had the privilege of teaching "Joc din Rebrisoara," a Romanian circle dance, and it was a special moment for us. On another occasion, Mr. Hagi was teaching a square dance. He had prepared several index cards with detailed instructions, and it took nearly an hour and a half to go through the steps before we were ready to dance to the music. To our surprise, it turned out to be a square dance with calls in English. Lothar and I, familiar with the calls, realized that the dance wasn't quite as complicated as it had seemed. Mr. Hagi, who doesn't speak English, had written down instructions from watching the dance on YouTube. While we had been dancing the correct figures, no one recognized the pattern until we heard the English calls. The dance was "Six Pass Thru." After we gently explained the meaning of the calls, the group was able to follow along with our cues.

Another memorable experience was when Mr. Hagi took us to a large festival in Ube, where we danced throughout the day. In the morning, we tried our best to keep up with dances we didn't know, making every effort not to embarrass our dance circle, which was important since we were representing them at the festival. It was quite exhausting. In the early afternoon, we were relieved to finally recognize two dances on the program: "Ya Da Kalinushku Lomala," a Russian dance, and "Adama Veshamayim," a dance from Israel. Thinking we could now relax a bit, we were caught off guard when, for "Ya Da Kalinushku Lomala," we were handed triangular scarves to hold between the leader and the follower, turning the familiar circle dance into a couple's dance with intricate patterns. Then came "Adama Veshamayim," and everything seemed familiar at first. But when the music sped up, it suddenly switched to a techno-rap beat. Lothar and I thought there must have been a glitch in the sound system, but to our amazement, all the other dancers carried on as if nothing had changed, continuing with the usual steps. It turned out this was simply how the dance was performed in that region.

Japan was full of unexpected and delightful surprises. More to come in the next chapter of our adventures.

7

Folk Dancing in Rural Japan: More Surprises

During our time in Japan, my son Lothar and I had the opportunity to participate in various folk dance events, including a daylong festival, weekly dance circles, and the Yamaguchi Summer Camp. At the camp's opening ceremony, roughly 170 participants lined up according to their registration numbers. Several people gave speeches, and I had been warned that I would be expected to give one too, simply because I was from the United States. Standing before such a large audience, I delivered the short speech I had prepared in Japanese, which was admittedly a bit nerve-wracking. Afterward, everyone sang the Yamaguchi Folk Dance Federation anthem, and Lothar and I were surprised to discover that such an anthem even existed! The lyrics spoke of the joy of folk dancing, followed by a series of "la-la-las."

Along with Bianca de Jong, a teacher from the Netherlands, Lothar and I were treated as VIPs, including a special lunch. Bianca taught an Azerbaijani dance called Bahar, which we loved so much that we brought it back to California and taught it at Changs. Her advice while teaching stuck with me: "If you make a mistake, make it in an elegant way!" When we taught Bahar at Changs, I passed on her words, but then, just two minutes later, I made a mistake and reacted in a far less elegant manner! Clearly, some lessons take time to sink in.

After the camp, Lothar and I traveled across Honshu, Japan's main island. Our first stop was Himeji in Hyogo Prefecture, not for its famous white castle but for an all-day folk dance workshop with Bulgarian teacher Ventsi Sotirov. We then visited my host family in Okazaki, Aichi Prefecture, where I had stayed for a month several years earlier. Eager to retain the dances we had just learned, we practiced everywhere: in their lovely garden, on a wooden platform in a park, and even near the top of a mountain while hiking. As we continued our journey, we reviewed the dances in our hotel rooms. Given the small size of most Japanese hotel rooms, we had to make do with a space barely 25 to 30 inches wide, just the length of the bed.

Sharing our passion for folk dancing with my Okazaki host family had a ripple effect. My host mother, Kumiko, was inspired to find a local folk dance group. Our conversations with her even led to a folk dance performance two years later. As a piano teacher, Kumiko invited us to her student's recital, where she asked us to demonstrate folk dancing at the end. Lothar and I couldn't showcase just one dance, as we wanted to convey the wonderful variety of international folk dances. So, we created a three-minute medley that included "Metzuit Acharet" from Israel, "Cimpoi" from Romania, "W moim Ogrodecku" from Poland, and "Nanban Ondo" from Japan. After our performance, we invited the students, all middle-schoolers, to join us on stage and dance "Savila Se Bela Loza" from Serbia. Of course, we had rehearsed everything beforehand.

As I mentioned in my speech at the Yamaguchi Summer Camp, my stay in Japan may not have improved my Japanese language skills as much as

I had hoped, but it certainly enriched my folk dancing experience.

8

Folk Dancing in a Buddhist Temple in Japan

During our stay at the Buddhist temple in Yamaguchi, Japan, I received the heartbreaking news that my dear friend and fellow folk dancer, Angel, had passed away unexpectedly. I was deeply shaken and overwhelmed with grief. Our host mother, Masumi, and her husband, the temple's head priest, provided immense comfort during this difficult time. The priest spoke with Lothar and me about the Buddhist perspective on death, gave us prayer beads, and performed a special Buddhist ceremony in honor of my friend. He also graciously allowed us to use the main temple for a folk dance session dedicated to Angel's memory. We coordinated with friends at Changs in San Francisco so that we could dance in her honor simultaneously—7:30 p.m. on Friday in California and 12:30 p.m. on Saturday in Japan. The priest borrowed my phone to play the music through the temple's sound system. It was early July, and the heat was intense. Lothar and I danced and cried for half an hour before the lack of air conditioning forced us to stop. Dancing to Angel's favorite songs brought us some comfort during that emotional time.

Now, let's move on to a more uplifting event. In addition to the temple's monthly open house, they occasionally hosted special events for the local community. During our stay, they organized a daylong workshop aimed at helping singles find partners. Around 30 young people attended. Masumi asked Lothar and me to teach them some folk dances, and we happily agreed, selecting a playlist of couple mixers we thought would be perfect for the occasion. We chose "T' Smidje," "La Bastringue,' and a charming dance called 'Harukaze no Yuwaku' (Spring Breeze Temptation). We prepared diligently, focusing on how best to teach folk dancing to beginners—all in Japanese, of course!

On the day of the event, we thought we were ready for anything. Masumi announced the folk dance portion, and the men lined up on one side of the room, the women on the other. However, when we asked them to form couples, no one moved! We tried rephrasing our instructions, but nothing changed. Masumi stepped in, encouraging everyone to pair off—one man with one woman—but still, no one budged. The men and women stood as far apart as possible, eyes downcast. Sensing our growing concern, Masumi finally took one woman by the hand and walked her over to the first man, breaking the ice. Slowly, they began to form couples, and we were able to teach the dances. Despite the initial challenge, the event turned out to be a lot of fun. We had anticipated difficulties with the dance steps, but never imagined that simply getting people to form couples would be the hardest part!

In an earlier chapter, I mentioned that the Buddhist temple hosted a monthly open house. In preparation for the first one after our arrival, our host mother Masumi invited a close friend who owns a beauty salon in nearby Tokuyama to come over. Her friend gave me a lovely set of gel nails and styled my hair, while Lothar's hair was arranged in a more traditional Japanese fashion. Soon after, a prominent local woman, an expert in kimono, arrived with her assistant. They provided traditional

Japanese attire for both of us and helped us dress—marking the first time in my adult life that someone had dressed me!

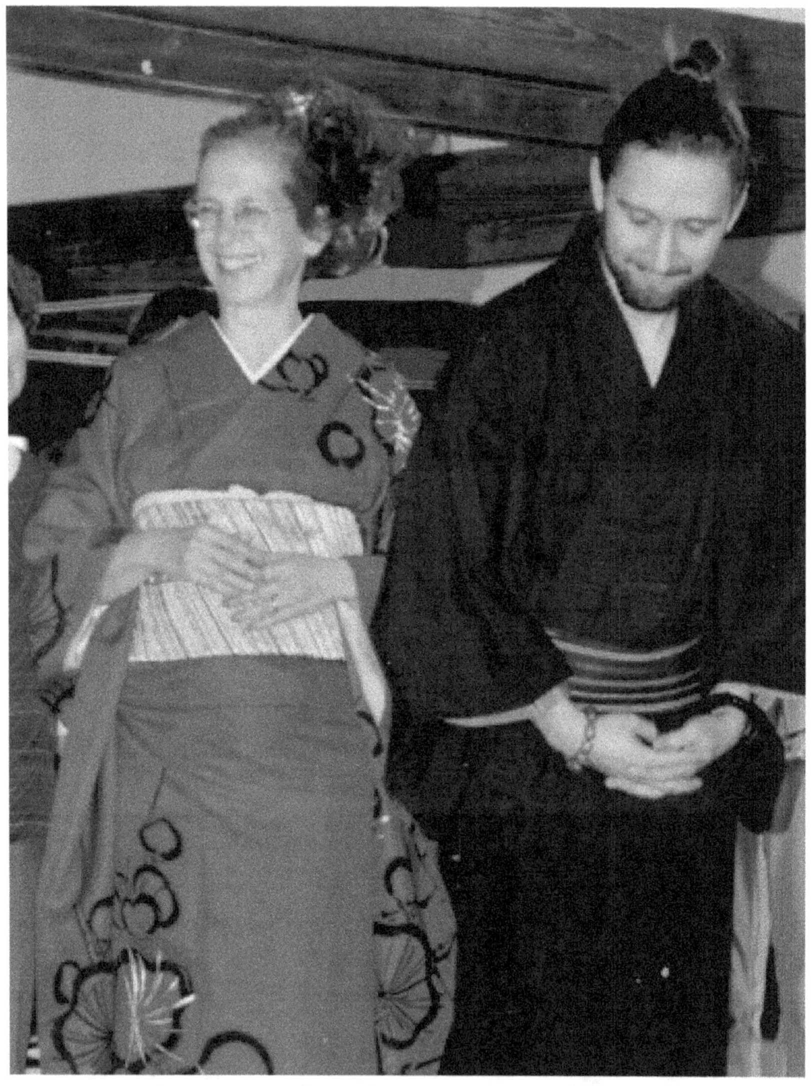

Lothar and me in our kimonos at the temple

We had invited local folk dancers to join us, but before dancing with them, Lothar and I performed two dances for all the guests. Dancing in unfamiliar outfits and in such a unique setting was an extraordinary experience. We chose "Liljano Mome" from Bulgaria and "Sharem El Sheikh" from Israel for our performance. Afterward, Mr. Hagi asked us to teach "Sharem El Sheikh" to his dance groups, which we happily did.

As our six-month stay drew to a close, our host family organized an unforgettable farewell party. They kept most of the details a surprise, only mentioning that they had invited some folk dancers, including the president of the Yamaguchi Folk Dance Federation. To express our gratitude, Lothar and I prepared two dances to perform: the Ukrainian dance "Holubka" and the Mexican dance "La Yaguesita," the latter requiring a hat for the leader and a fan for the follower.

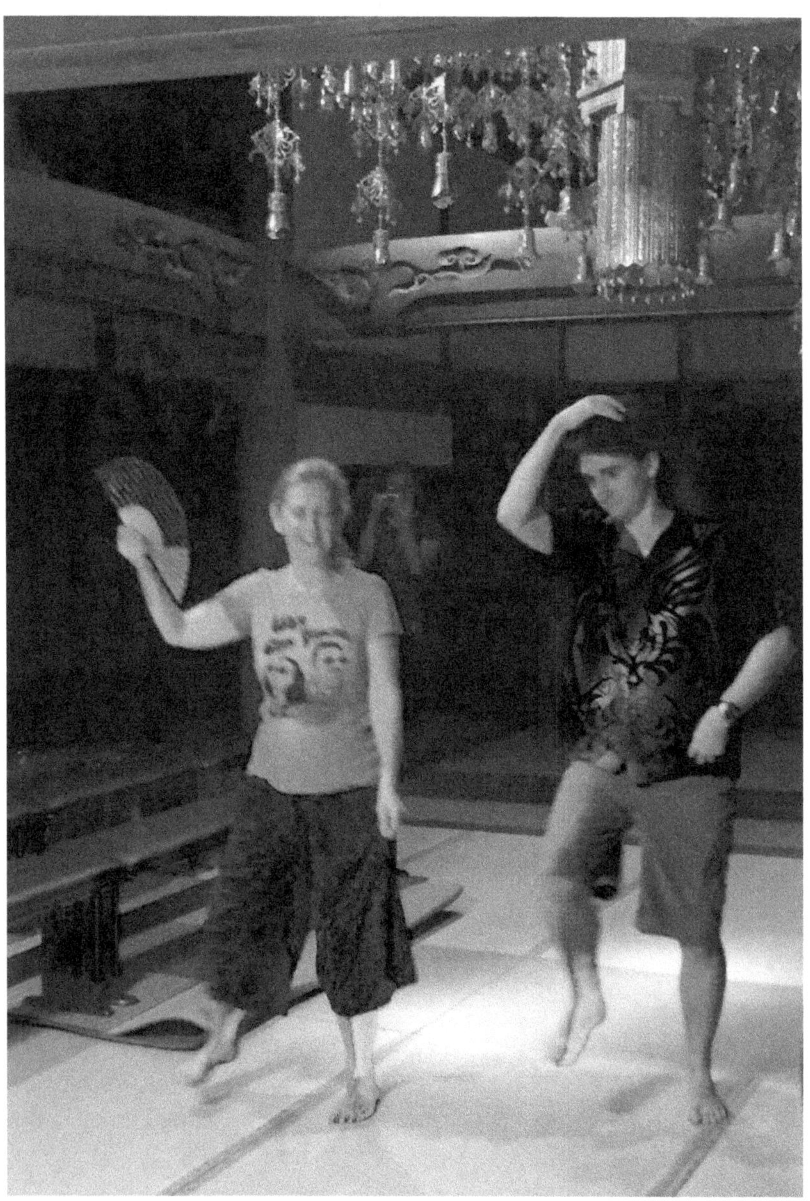

Me and Lothar dancing "La Yaguesita"

Naturally, there was also some folk dancing, not only with the folk dancers but with all the other guests as well.

One of the surprises at the party was a "noodle slide" that they had built in the backyard. Using bamboo halves laid end to end, with the hollow side facing up, the slide was tilted so that noodles and water could be released from the top. Guests lined up along the slide, trying to catch the noodles with chopsticks as they flowed down. Whatever noodles weren't caught ended up in a pot at the bottom. When the noodles ran out, they switched to grapes, which were much trickier to grab with chopsticks! The celebration also featured a large banner with well-wishes, a mini-concert, gifts, speeches, fireworks, and a singalong.

Folk dancing truly creates a sense of community, bringing together people who love to share joyful moments. Our folk dance activities added so much fun and connection to the lives of those in and around the temple.

9

The Importance of Music in Folk Dance

In the February 2024 issue of *Let's Dance!* one part of the article "Why I Started Folk Dancing" truly struck a chord with me: "The music played, and my body began to move in time with it. At that moment, as I felt my body follow the rhythm and flow with the music, I was hooked..." Indeed, the music in folk dancing is crucial to my experience. I remember when "Cetvorno," a Bulgarian dance from Yves Moreau, was taught in one of the classes I attended. At the time, I was still too new to master the steps, but the music captivated me so much that I later made the effort to learn the dance. My son Lothar slowed down the music significantly to help me grasp the rhythm. The exhilaration I felt when the music finally guided my feet was unforgettable.

Several years later, "Cetvorno" was included in the playlist at a dance event. While the steps were the same, the music had changed, and it didn't resonate with me at all. For that version, I would never have gone through the trouble of learning the dance.

Similarly, Greek dances were a mystery to me in my early years of folk dancing. I couldn't feel the rhythm, and it felt mechanical, as if I were just trying to match the steps of more experienced dancers. Only after years of practice did I begin to hear the beat in Greek music, and with that, the dances became far more enjoyable.

There were times when we learned a dance with a complex rhythm that I struggled to master, leading me to decide I didn't like the dance. But if it captivated Lothar, I'd give it another try. And when that moment finally came, when the music connected with my body and the movement flowed naturally, it was exhilarating and I changed my mind about this dance.

For many dances, there are at least two versions of the music, or an alternative piece is available. It's essential for me to find the version that makes me want to dance. Recently, I rediscovered the music for "Ketri Ketri" that Lothar and I had brought back from Japan. I found it much more exciting than the one in our Changs' music library, and I became obsessed with it for about a week, dancing "Ketri Ketri" to this newfound version at every opportunity—even while waiting for the tea water to boil.

When I fall in love with a piece of music, I often wish there was a dance to go with it, and sometimes I discover that one exists. That recently happened with "Despacito". And then there's "Conquest of Paradise" by Vangelis, the main theme of the movie "1492." I've always loved that music and never imagined it could have a dance. But at Stockton in 2023, Richard Powers played a modified version of "Conquest of Paradise" for a cross-step waltz, and I was in heaven—finally, I could dance to that music!

I am deeply grateful that my life is filled with this beautiful union of music and movement, also known as dance!

10

Folk Dance: A Gateway to Cultural Understanding

There are so many things I love about folk dancing. Of course, the music, the rhythms, the joy of movement, and the mental and physical challenge of learning new dances all hold a special place in my heart. The sense of accomplishment when I finally master a dance that once felt impossible is incredibly fulfilling.

Equally, I cherish the wonderful people I've met along the way and the warm, welcoming atmosphere that surrounds the folk dancing community.

But there is another dimension to folk dancing that I deeply value, one that isn't often discussed. Over the years, folk dancing has given me profound insights into diverse cultures—lessons I never would have encountered otherwise.

For example, in some regions, people form closed circles while dancing, believing it keeps evil spirits out. In other cultures, open circles are preferred, allowing negative spirits to escape. Some traditions embrace a heavy, grounded style of dancing to reflect their connection to the earth, while others feature dancers standing tall and proud. In yet other places, the movements are quick and light, embodying a different kind of energy.

In some cultures, dancers shout or make loud noises while they move, while in others, silence is an essential part of the experience. There are places where men and women dance separately at times, and in some traditions, such separation is unthinkable.

In certain dances, the order of dancers in an open circle is of great significance.

Absorbing these cultural nuances wasn't about memorizing facts for me. It was a different kind of learning, one that came naturally through experience. I no longer remember all the details, but what has stayed with me is a powerful lesson: there isn't one "right" way of doing things. There are many ways, and all of them are valid.

This understanding reaches far beyond dance. It applies to every aspect of life. The way people do things—how they think, live, and solve problems—is neither better nor worse in my family, my neighborhood, or my country than it is elsewhere. It's simply different.

Folk dancing has opened my mind to other perspectives, making me less judgmental and more curious about the lives of others. I am eager to learn in ways I hadn't imagined before.

And to think I once believed folk dancing was just about fancy footwork!

11

Awareness of Space

I will address a subject close to my heart—namely, the sometimes less than ideal communal awareness in dance. I'm talking about people's sense of space, which is to say their awareness of their surroundings and their relationship with fellow dancers.

Have you ever noticed how, just before a dance begins, people form a large circle, cramming together on one side while the other side remains sparsely populated? This imbalance can be amusing, but it highlights a certain disconnection in our collective experience. The dance, after all, is not solely about the individual; it is a shared moment that thrives on mutual respect and awareness.

Occasionally someone will dance a bit to the inside of the circle for a better view of the feet of a dancer a few places ahead of them. This makes the circle resemble a crooked potato.

Then, when a dance ends, what happens? A cluster of chatty dancers decides to have an impromptu get-together right on the dance floor. Whoever wants to do the next dance must pull off an elaborate maneuver to avoid collisions.

Every so often someone in the line will hold your hand a bit too tightly. It's a reminder that we're not always in tune with our neighbors.

When people hold hands while dancing, the circle can widen to the point where one's arms are extended too far, which feels uncomfortable. In this situation, all dancers can step toward the center of the circle to bring everyone closer. And if this does not help or the dancer is not aware of this possibility, he or she might be forced to break the line just to seek relief.

Another crucial aspect of awareness arises when dancers are behind the lines trying to learn the steps. If there's not enough space between the dancers and the wall or chairs, it becomes rather cramped, especially when people need to do turns. If the people in the main line or circle don't pay attention, there could be collisions or the people behind the lines will not have a pleasant dance experience.

When I danced in Japan, I noticed a marked difference in how people related to one another on the dance floor. The circles were rounder and more evenly spaced—no awkward potatoes in sight—and everyone seemed attuned to the harmony of the group. This isn't surprising, considering that in Japanese culture maintaining group harmony is often prioritized over individual expression. By contrast, here in the United States, and maybe also in other western countries, our culture emphasizes individual rights and personal freedom, which can sometimes lead to a lack of awareness about how our actions affect those around us.

I want to encourage mindfulness. Let's become more aware of our surroundings and how our movements affect one another. As we dance together, let's strive for balance. It's wonderful to express ourselves and enjoy our individual moments, but let's also remember the joy of moving together. After all, dancing is not just about the steps; it's also about the connection we build with one another in that shared space.

12

Folk Dance costumes

When Lothar and I lived in a Buddhist temple in Yamaguchi Prefecture, Japan, for an extended period, we danced with local groups every week. As I mentioned in an earlier chapter, at first, the dancers were a bit shy and nervous around us, but after several weeks, we all grew more comfortable with one another. This was especially noticeable in how the women responded to my attire. I typically wore simple pants or a basic skirt with a blouse or T-shirt to our dance evenings, while most of the other women dressed in more elaborate clothing, specific to folk dancing. One evening, a woman approached me before the dancing started and gave me a two-part dress that resembled the other women's outfits. I immediately changed into it and danced, but I quickly realized that the dress was far too hot. The following week, another woman brought me a white blouse with embroidered details and a skirt similar to theirs. When I wore that blouse the next time the folk dancers visited the temple, two women pulled me aside, insisting that I had put it on backward. They helped me turn it around, only for us to realize that the blouse was perfectly symmetrical! Despite the mix-up, I was deeply touched by their care and attention.

I had heard that, in the "old days," if you wanted to join Changs International Folk Dancers in San Francisco, you were expected to bring your own folk dance costume. When I started folk dancing in 2009, quite a few women still wore folk dance outfits, dresses, or skirts to dance. But in recent years, most people seem to dance in casual clothes. Similarly, ethnic dress was more common at parties in the past, but now it's a rare sight.

Before I joined the folk dance community, I wasn't particularly fond of traditional Austrian garments. But being exposed to so many different cultures has given me a new appreciation for my own traditions. I even acquired a Dirndl from the region where I was born, and I now wear it for special dance occasions.

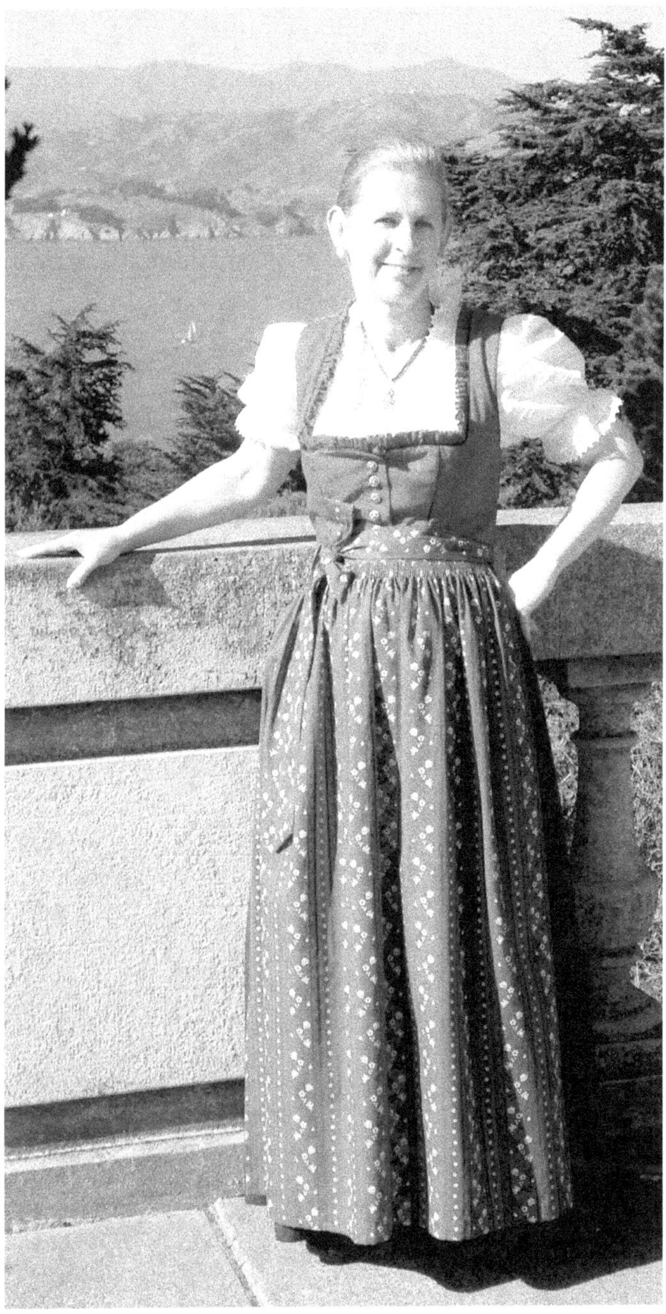

Me in my Dirndl

I must admit, though, that I'm grateful no one judges me for dancing in casual clothes. My ideal dance outfit is one that allows me to climb a ladder to help with decorations, makes it easy for people to see my feet when I lead a dance, and is practical enough to keep me warm if I step outside or cool enough to keep me comfortable while dancing. It takes a special effort for me to get dressed up, and that mood only strikes a few times a year.

However, one memorable experience has given me a strong reason to dress up occasionally and contribute to the festive atmosphere of a folk dance event. It happened in 2018 at Stockton Folk Dance Camp, during the "Wednesday Romani Rumble." As I entered the dance hall, everyone was dancing Dana, a Romanian Roma dance, and the sight of all the colorful, swirling skirts completely covering the floor was a breathtaking moment, one that I will never forget.

13

Folk Dancing on Zoom

I'm still filled with joy that, with the pandemic behind us, we can once again dance together in person. Now that the heated debates over "to Zoom or not to Zoom" have settled, I feel ready to share my experiences with Zoom dancing.

On March 13, 2020, Changs International Folk Dancers held its regular Friday evening dance, but in an effort to prevent the spread of the new virus, we decided not to hold hands. We were practicing for the Blossom Festival scheduled for late April, confident that everything would be back to normal by then! But on March 16, a stay-at-home order was issued for San Francisco, and as we now know, it would be much longer before life returned to normal. The Blossom Festival didn't happen that year—or the next.

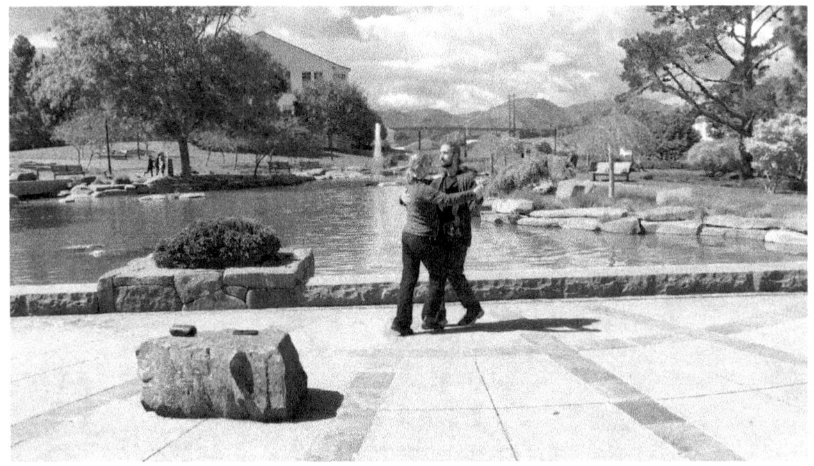

Lothar and me dancing in the Presidio by the pond near our favorite Starbucks

The thought of not dancing was unbearable, so my son Lothar and I started dancing outdoors. We began at the Presidio by the pond near our favorite Starbucks, then moved to Eagles Point at the Lands End trailhead. We tried dancing in an alcove in the Lands End parking lot before finally discovering our favorite spot—near the Legion of Honor, next to the fountain.

We also participated in various Zoom dance events, like those hosted by the Palomanians or Udy Gold, joining in from our living room. But soon I began missing my folk dance friends from Changs, so Lothar and I explored the possibility of hosting our own Zoom dance events. On June 12, 2020, we did just that for the first time, and it became a regular occurrence. We would dance for 90 minutes, followed by a "social hour" with a different theme and moderator each week.

These Zoom gatherings added a new dimension to our dance experience. We got to know each other much better—when someone spoke, everyone listened, a change from in-person events where the music would often interrupt conversations, drawing people to the dance floor mid-sentence.

We learned fascinating things about each other during show-and-tell evenings. Before the dances, Lothar and I shared videos of Scottish and English set dances we couldn't perform on Zoom, as well as clips of our own dancing in Japan or quirky dance-related findings, such as the dance sequence in the 1966 sci-fi show "Raumpatrouille Orion". (Look it up on YouTube: search for "Raumpatrouille Orion Ep 01," and watch from 9:55 to 11:30). Dancers joined us from Southern California, Washington State, and beyond—people who knew Changs dancers from Stockton, the annual Folk Dance Camp, though some had never visited Changs itself. We even watched one dancer interact with her cat, who insisted on being held during the dances, jumping up until she was scooped into her arms!

When I visited my sister in Austria, Zoom allowed me to stay connected to the Changs dancers. I'd get up at 4 a.m., put on headphones connected to my cell phone, and quietly dance around the bed in the dark to avoid waking my brother.

Dancing in our living room, however, was quite a challenge. It's a small space, especially for two dancers. During our first attempt at "Tfilati," an Israeli dance that features a lot of turning, I painfully caught my fingers in Lothar's while turning. We also found it disorienting, as the "center" of the dance for each of us wasn't the middle of the room but a point on the opposite side of our circle. For example, in "Libi," you walk toward the center, turn halfway, and face outward—where I would see Lothar directly across from me. Dancing "Libi" in a much larger space in person was a revelation; when I turned and faced out, there was no one looking back at me!

We adapted some dances to fit the small space. For "Jacob's Ladder," an Israeli circle dance, we didn't hold hands but danced facing each other, and the box step became a do-si-do[1]. For "Shir Al Etz," an Israeli dance in an open circle, we made only a half-turn instead of a full turn before the last part of the dance, which meant taking turns leading.

On February 25, 2022, Lothar and I hosted our last Zoom dance session, and the following week, Changs resumed in-person dancing at our new location.

I believe that many in the dance community found creative ways to embrace Zoom, making those years of confinement and social distancing feel far less isolating.

---

[1] do-si-do: a figure in which two dancers pass around each other back to back and return to their original positions

14

When leaders go on vacation

As mentioned previously, when Lothar and I lived at a Buddhist temple in Yamaguchi Prefecture for an extended period, we danced with local groups each week. One group, led by Mr. Hagi, consisted entirely of women. He would arrive early before each dance evening to practice the dances he had prepared. At the exact start time, he would lead the group through warm-up exercises, followed by the teaching of several dances. Over the next two or three weeks, he would review those dances with the group before introducing new ones.

During a two-week period when Mr. Hagi returned to his hometown, the group was left without a leader, and I was intrigued to see how things changed. Several women stepped up to teach dances they wanted to share, bringing their own music and helping each other with the instructions. The atmosphere became much more relaxed, with plenty of laughter and joking. However, when Mr. Hagi returned, the mood returned to its usual seriousness.

A similar situation occurred last year at our San Francisco folk dance club. Three of our dance leaders, including myself, were out of town, leaving the group to manage on its own. During those leaderless evenings, many people took turns leading the dances, or the group collectively figured out the steps. They reported, with great joy, that the announcement time had shrunk to just 30 seconds, allowing them to fit in 42 dances—a truly fun experience!

About ten years ago, a different scenario played out at our club. While the main teacher and several experienced dancers were attending Stockton Folk Dance Camp, the rest of us tried to get through a dance session on our own. At that time, I was still a beginner and couldn't lead any dances. We played beautiful music and moved about, but it was mostly an aimless, confused attempt—grapevines and step-lifts here and there, but not much real dancing. We eagerly awaited the return of our dance leaders.

From these experiences, I've learned a few things. It's valuable for everyone to know how to lead at least a few dances. It might also be beneficial for experienced dance leaders to occasionally join the line of dancers in the middle or wait until someone else has started leading before joining. Stepping out of the leading position after one or two repetitions of the dance and joining the end of the line could also help ease a less-experienced dancer into leading.

15

Embarrassing Moments

My most embarrassing moment occurred in 2017. That spring, I attended the Ontario Folk Dance Camp, where I learned a version of the Greek dance "Rododachtilos." Feeling confident, I volunteered to teach it at the Summer Camps Review in Palo Alto and submitted the music and dance description in advance.

On the day of the workshop, the heat was intense. During lunch, I helped unload the organizer's car, making several trips between the car and the dance hall under the blazing sun. When the reviews began, I sat through the teaching of 10 dances before my turn. Exhausted from lack of sleep, overwhelmed by the heat, and trying to absorb those earlier dances, I felt mentally drained.

When it was finally my turn to teach "Rododachtilos," I began by explaining the first part, which was simple. But when I reached the second part, which was just a basic grapevine in Syrto rhythm, my mind went blank. I couldn't remember the steps, and my feet refused to cooperate. I was horrified, convinced that I had lost all respect from the folk dance community and that I might never be able to return.

Thankfully, another teacher stepped in to help, and somehow, the teaching session came to a close, although I can hardly recall how it ended. Afterwards, many people approached me to reassure me, sharing their own stories of similar moments and encouraging me not to worry. To my relief, not only did the community continue to welcome me, but I later even became president of the Folk Dance Federation!

Another time, I narrowly avoided an embarrassing situation. It happened at a workshop with Ira Weisburd, a well-known choreographer, at St. Bede's in Menlo Park. The workshop had ended, and during the party, the dance "Mori Shej" began. Ira was leading the line, starting with steps I didn't recognize. I was tempted to rush to the front and lead with the "correct" steps. Thankfully, I held back, and I'm so glad I did! It turned out that Ira was dancing a version choreographed by Laura Shannon for the first few repetitions, before switching to the one I knew by Jimmy Drury. Ira had been teaching "Mori Shej" that way. Even if he had been "wrong," it wouldn't have been appropriate for me to take over. That moment taught me to respect the leader's role and that it's poor form to interfere.

I am truly grateful that the folk dance family is so forgiving and supportive.

16

Stockton Folk Dance Camps: Cherished Memories

Before I share just why our times at camp were so fantastic, let me tell you about a few challenges we faced.

- It is always tough to get up after naps, with my sleep-deprived body begging for more rest. But the events awaiting me were so exciting that I never once extended my nap time.
- We learned some incredibly difficult dances, but the sense of accomplishment and joy after finally mastering their complex rhythms made all the effort more than worthwhile.
- And, of course, saying goodbye to dear friends at the end of camp was hard. Yet, parting also meant the beginning of joyful anticipation for next year's reunion.

On Wednesdays at Stockton, there's a Candle Lighting Ceremony to welcome new dancers into the Stockton Folk Dance family. When I attended Stockton Folk Dance Camp for the first time, my fellow dancers from Changs stood beside me in a darkened room as the candles were lit. I was deeply touched by the moment and felt an overwhelming sense of inclusion and welcome, far exceeding my expectations. As the candlelight song played, tears of gratitude streamed down my face.

In one of my first years at camp, Caspar Bik was teaching "Rashovda," a dance he created using traditional Georgian steps. Over the course of the week, he taught us the various figures to slowed-down music. It wasn't until Friday that we danced the entire sequence at full speed. "Rashovda" was particularly challenging for me, yet to my amazement, I managed to perform it at full speed. That Friday night, during the evening review session, I was filled with pure joy while dancing "Rashovda." The love of that music and that magical moment have stayed with me ever since.

At one Stockton Folk Dance Camp, we learned the dance "Firetur" in Richard Powers' class. This lively dance involves two couples dancing with each other. One figure, called the "Arm Hook," has the leader hook right elbows with the follower of the other couple for a clockwise turn. The leaders then pass each other back to back, hook left elbows with their own partner for two counter-clockwise turns, and finally switch back to the other couple's follower. The switching part was the trickiest aspect of the dance. The first time we danced it to music, the switch didn't go as planned. The woman from the other couple accidentally hit me in the face with her fist while trying to reach the other leader. It hurt, but we all laughed and kept dancing. The next time around, we mastered the switch perfectly!

The talent show was a celebration of all kinds of performances, from dancing and singing to playing instruments, putting on a comedic game show, and reciting poetry. It was all delightful. When I mentioned this to a friend, she asked, "Who won?" That made me realize—there are no winners or losers at Stockton, just a joyful sharing of talents.

During one talent show, Adony, the tech guy of the day, shared a video of a past performance where Vicky U. showcased her poi ball skills, which was fitting since that year the Polynesian teacher Kau'i had been teaching us how to use them. As we watched the video projected onto a big screen, everything seemed fine until the screen went black, displaying a message like "waiting for input signal." Adony didn't notice that we couldn't see the video and kept watching his laptop, completely entertained and laughing uproariously. It was almost more fun for us to watch him than the video itself! Eventually, he figured it out, found a new cable, and showed us the whole clip.

For another talent show, my son Lothar and I worked with four other couples to learn the "Russian Suite." During rehearsals, we had several moments where the dance could have turned into a comedy routine, but we kept it poised and elegant. The performance went smoothly, and we were just about to bow when the music suddenly stopped, and without warning or pause, a lively, upbeat tune began—completely contrasting with the slow, dignified Russian music we had been dancing to. Unable to bow or leave the stage as planned, we laughed along with the audience and made a chaotic exit, turning our graceful routine into an unintended comedy after all!

At Stockton Richard Powers shared insightful lectures with us, similar to those he gives his students at Stanford, about the essence of social dancing. He emphasized that focusing on others, especially your partner, enriches the experience of any couple dance. In a dance class, it's natural to want your partner to do the steps correctly to help you learn, and you might be tempted to critique or guide them. While it's acceptable to gently point out mistakes when learning new steps, once we start dancing, our mindset should shift. We should treat our partner as the most important person at that moment, delight in the time spent together, and strive to make their dance experience as enjoyable as possible. I took Richard's words to heart and felt a sense of exhilaration when I applied them. I stopped obsessing over getting the steps perfect and instead smiled at my partner, grateful for those few shared minutes, adjusting my movements to ensure a smoother dance. This shift felt liberating and deepened my connection with my dance partner.

In Željko Jergan's class, we learned "Goričani," a Croatian dance known for its unique middle finger hold. Instead of clasping hands or pinkies, dancers interlock their middle fingers. After Stockton, while driving home from a coffee shop, I found myself behind a driver who angrily rolled down his window and stuck out his middle finger at another driver. This sparked an amusing idea—how to defuse a similar situation if anyone ever gave me the finger. I could simply smile and say, "Oh yes, I know that dance too!" I hope I never have to test if this approach would actually work!

17

Memorable Dance Moments: An A-to-Z Journey

When we dance, we enjoy the movement, the music, the sense of accomplishment, and the company of our fellow dancers. We also associate certain dances with both interesting moments and cherished experiences. I would like to present those kinds of memories from my life as a folk dancer, and I'll do so in alphabetical order.

Ba La (Israeli mixer): While discussing something with my son Lothar, I responded to his comment with an emotional "Ay-ay-ay!" He immediately started singing "ay-ay-ay" as it is sung in one of our dances, but we could not figure out which one it was. The next time we went to Changs, we asked Craig Blackstone, our teacher, for the name of the dance. After thinking for a bit, he told us it was "Ba La." The "ay-ay-ay" comes two minutes into the dance.

Besof Ma'agal (Israeli couple dance): I had a hard time remembering the name of this dance until Lothar came up with a funny way. The German word "besoffen" means "drunk," and "mir egal" means "I don't care."

So "Besof Ma'agal" sounds like "Besoffen? Mir egal!" which would mean "Drunk? I don't care!"

Ciuleandra (Open circle dance from Romania): Whenever we dance this, I hear Craig's singing, "She forgot the baby eggs" or "She forgot to lay the eggs." Although this is a Romanian song, some parts sound similar to the above English words. If you want to see the whole song interpreted as English, go to YouTube and type in *"She forgot to lay the eggs" – Ciuleandra misheard lyrics* in the search box.

De Valse Zeeman (The Netherlands, couples in a circle): When I learned this dance, I saw Angel turning in the first pattern while holding her left hand behind her back. I thought that that was what all followers should do. When I checked with her, she said she was just holding her long braid so it wouldn't whip someone's face as she turned!

Hora Nuntasilor (Open circle dance from Romania): I vividly remember the late Laila Messer leading this dance. In fact, at Changs we call it "Laila's dance." With great enthusiasm, she always grabbed her husband or a newcomer to join the line.

Kvar Acharey Hatzot (open circle dance from Israel): During our last dance of the night, Udy Gold, the teacher of our Israeli dance class, explained what each line of this poetic song means in English. Then he reached the part that goes, "Tomorrow it will be another day / And what can you expect from a new day?" At that point someone interjected, "Olivia's colonoscopy!" (Name changed to protect the privacy)

Libi (Israel): This is the song where I had the privilege to witness the "finding" of two words in the lyrics that sound like something we know, one is "Vallejo" and the other is "Escargot." Now I sing along when

"Vallejo" or "Escargot" comes on.

Liljano Mome (Bulgaria, open circle): And here is another case of misheard lyrics. Toward the end of this song, we seem to hear "uvula" a lot!

Livavtini (Israeli couple dance): Lothar and I had learned both roles for some couple dances and experienced that this was quite hard. So, we had the idea of dancing this at Stockton's talent show and switching roles a few times. But when we tried it out, we found that it took no talent at all for this dance and was totally easy.

Oj devojko duso moja (open circle dance from Serbia): Lothar and I lived only two blocks away from the church where we danced each Friday night. In the early days of our folk dancing instead of walking home we sometimes danced this all the way home.

Oslo Waltz (England/Scotland mixer): I was still a very inexperienced dancer when I volunteered to be a leader. So far, I had only danced this dance as a follower where I always started by turning to the right and moving in front of the person to my right to land on his or her other side. Before the dance started, I repeated to myself, "I am a leader, I am a leader" to not forget to stand still and roll the follower from my left side to the right side. Then the music started and I immediately danced the follower's part! Darn!

Populli Jon (open circle dance from Albania): When I first saw this dance, Violet was leading it. The person to her side was much taller than she, so Violet held her arms way up high. I assumed that's what leaders were supposed to do, and for several months, whenever I led this dance I did the same thing, which was quite strenuous.

Shoofni (open circle dance from Israel): When I think of the name of this dance, I always hear a dear fellow dancer calling it "Shoot me!" We incorporated this joke into the medley when celebrating the 80th anniversary of Changs.

Trip to Hexham (English country dance for three couples): To teach this dance at the Ontario Folk Dance Camp, Anne Leach showed it with a demonstration set. Of the three leaders, one was a man. The female leaders had no distinguishing accessories, like a sash or a tie. At one point something went wrong, and the teacher stopped the dance and asked "Who are the men?" The one man timidly raised his hand, but none of the female leaders spoke up!

I hope this brings a smile to your face and helps you remember touching or funny moments when you are dancing.

18

Conclusion

Folk dancing brings enrichment to so many facets of life: physically, through the movement and energy it requires; mentally, as you challenge yourself to learn new dances; emotionally, as you're touched by the beauty of the music; and socially, as you connect with others while dancing in a vibrant community.

If you liked this book please take the time and leave a favorable review on Amazon!

19

Resources

I f you're looking for places to enjoy folk dancing in Northern California, click on the Community tab at *folkdance.com* and use the interactive map. You can find both in-person and virtual dance events.

For Southern California, explore local dance clubs through *SoCal Folk Dance.org*.

To find folk dance groups across the U.S., the National Folk Organization maintains a website, *nfo-usa.org,* where you will also find an interactive map under the Where to Dance tab.